Harry Goes to the
Hospital

For Coby, Sophie, and Josh – HJB

In memory of Walter Herbst – MSW

Published by
MAGINATION PRESS
An Educational Publishing Foundation Book
American Psychological Association
750 First Street, NE
Washington, DC 20002

For more information about our books, including a complete catalog, please write to us, call 1-800-374-2721, or visit our website at www.maginationpress.com.

Editor: Becky Shaw
Art Director: Susan K. White
Printed by Phoenix Color, Rockaway, New Jersey

Library of Congress Cataloging-in-Publication Data

Bennett, Howard J.
Harry goes to the hospital : a story for children about what it's like to be
in the hospital / by Howard J. Bennett ; illustrated by M.S. Weber.
p. cm.
ISBN-13: 978-1-4338-0319-2 (harcover : alk. paper)
ISBN-10: 1-4338-0319-4 (hardcover : alk. paper)
ISBN-13: 978-1-4338-0320-8 (pbk. : alk. paper)
ISBN-10: 1-4338-0320-8 (pbk. : alk. paper)
1. Children—Hospital care—Juvenile literature. 2. Sick children—Juvenile literature.
I. Weber, M.S. (Michael S.) ill. II. Title.
RJ242.B45 2008
362.198'92—dc22   2007039577

10 9 8 7 6 5 4 3 2 1

Harry Goes to the Hospital

**A Story for Children About
What It's Like to Be in the Hospital**

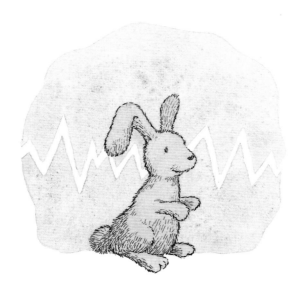

by Howard J. Bennett, M.D.
illustrated by M.S. Weber

MAGINATION PRESS • WASHINGTON, DC

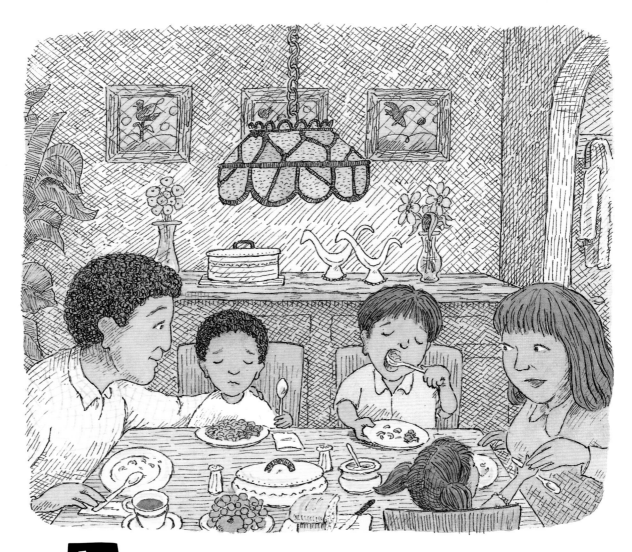

The night Harry got sick, his mom made his
favorite dinner—macaroni and cheese. Harry got a
tummy ache after one spoonful and told his mom he
wasn't hungry. She knew right away that something
was wrong because Harry wouldn't turn down
macaroni and cheese in a million years.

"Why don't you go upstairs and lie down?" she said.
"One of us will be up in a minute to check on you."

As soon as Harry got upstairs he started throwing up. He threw up so many times that it scared him because he had never done that before. His mom called the doctor to find out what to do. Dr. Walker said to take Harry to the hospital emergency room—that's where you go when you need to see a doctor right away!

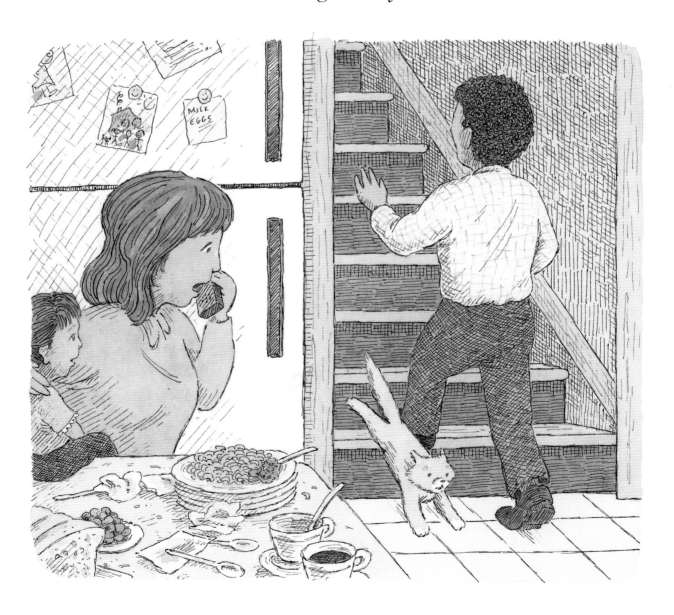

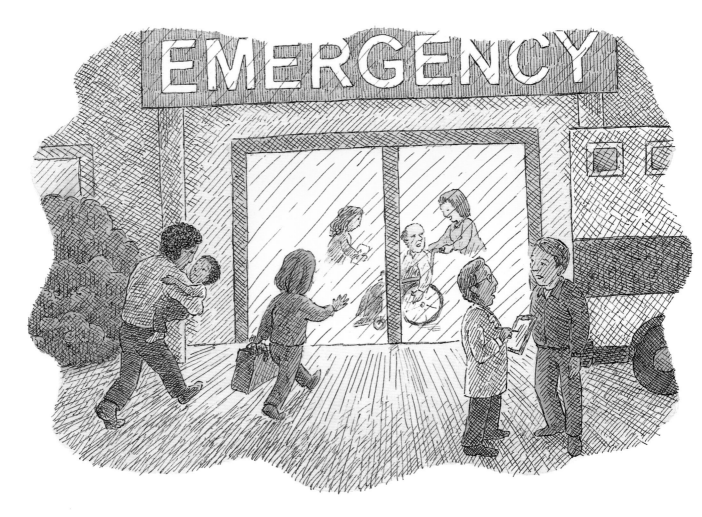

Harry had never been to a hospital and was scared about what would happen to him once he got there. His mom told him that the doctors and nurses would do everything they could to make him feel better.

Harry hugged his dad tightly. "Are you going to leave me there?" he asked.

"No, no of course not," his mom told him. "The doctors will give you some medicine to make your vomiting stop. Your dad or I will stay with you until you're okay." That made Harry feel a little better.

Once they got to
the emergency room,
the first person Harry
met was a nurse.

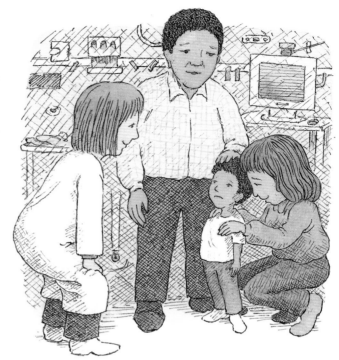

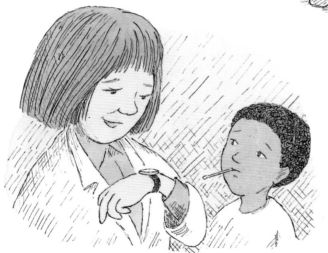

She weighed him and
took his temperature
just like the nurses did
at Dr. Walker's office.

She also gave
Harry a special
bracelet with his
name on it.

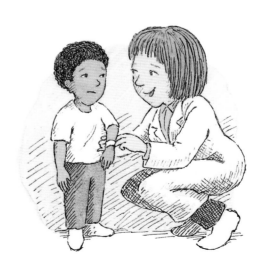

The emergency room was really busy. Doctors and nurses were running around. There were beeps and strange sounds coming from weird looking machines. Some of them reminded Harry of his older brother's video games. There were also lots of people in hospital beds. It was more sick people than Harry had ever seen. It made Harry feel kind of nervous, but his dad explained that these machines helped the doctors take care of the sick people.

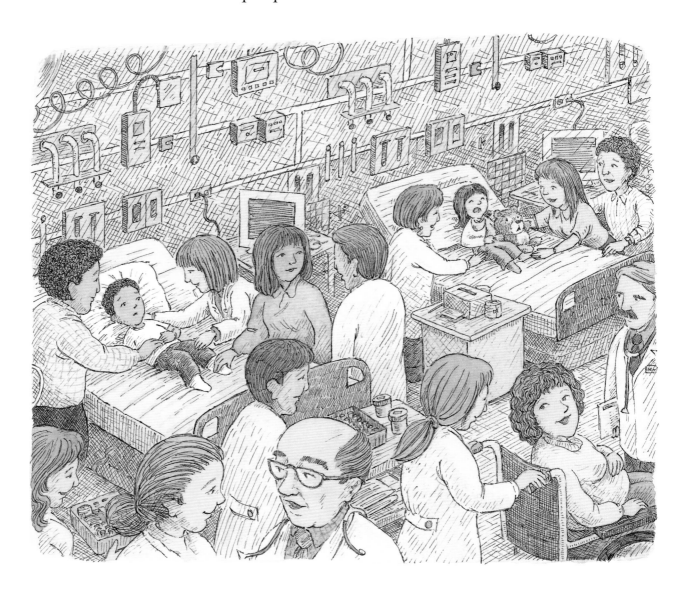

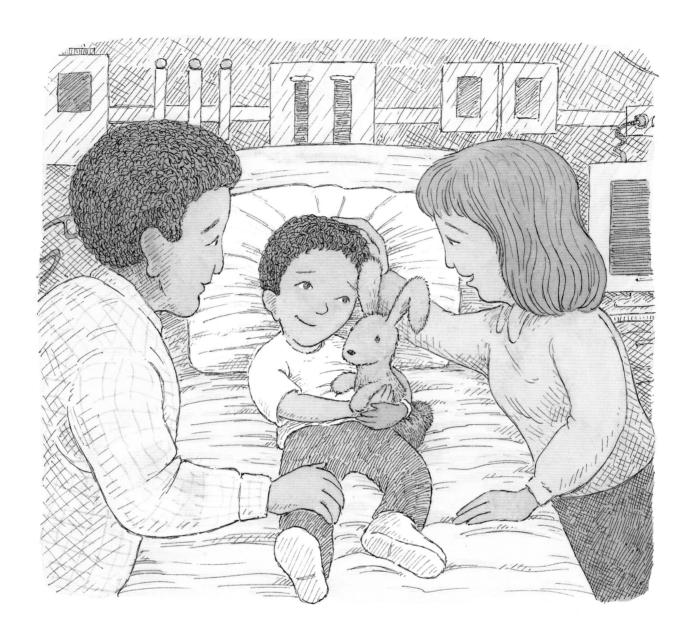

"Where's Barney?" Harry cried.
"Don't worry, he's right here,"
said his mom as she reached into
Harry's overnight bag.
Having Barney around always
made Harry feel better.

"Hello, Harry," said a woman with a big smile.

"My name is Dr. Meadows. I'm going to give you a checkup like your doctor does in his office."

Harry wasn't too sure he liked this new doctor. Dr. Walker always said hello to Barney and asked how he was feeling. So Harry's mom asked the doctor if she could check Barney too.

"Is Barney sick?" said Dr. Meadows as she gently pushed on his tummy.

Harry nodded his head and then looked down.

"I think maybe you and Barney have a bad case of stomach flu," she said. "Your body needs some water to make you better."

"How much do I have to drink?" asked Harry.

"Well, we don't want you to drink it because you'd probably throw up anything you swallow tonight. So we have to give you the water through a tiny needle in your arm called an IV."

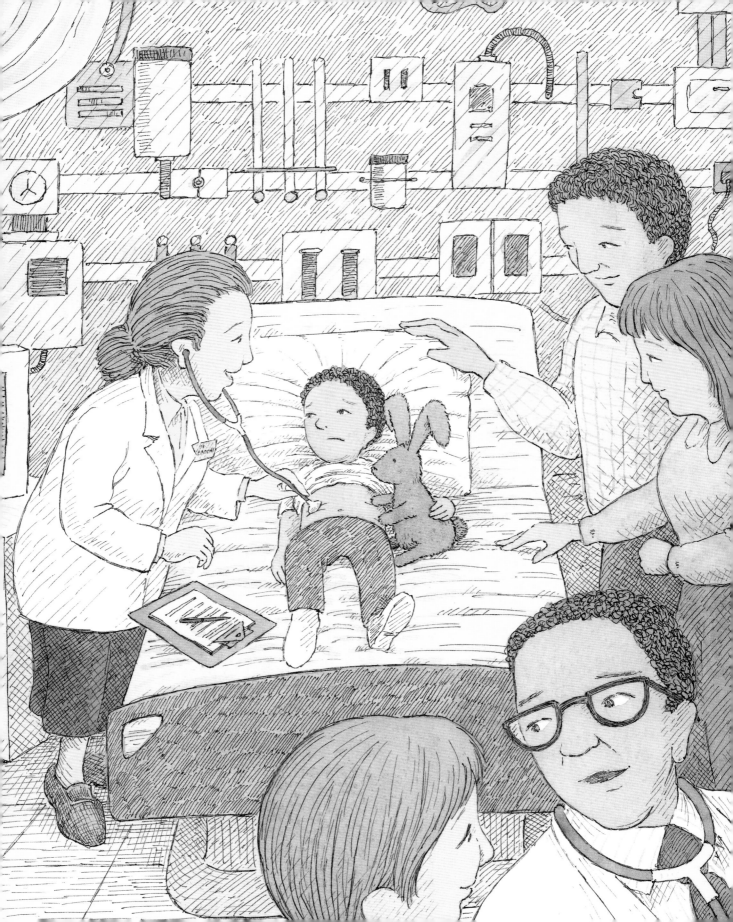

Harry hugged Barney tighter and started to cry. He told his mother he didn't need an IV, and he promised Dr. Meadows he wouldn't throw up anymore. Harry hated all the new things that were happening. He just wanted to go home.

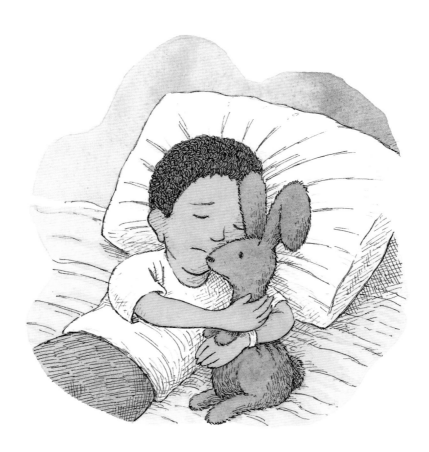

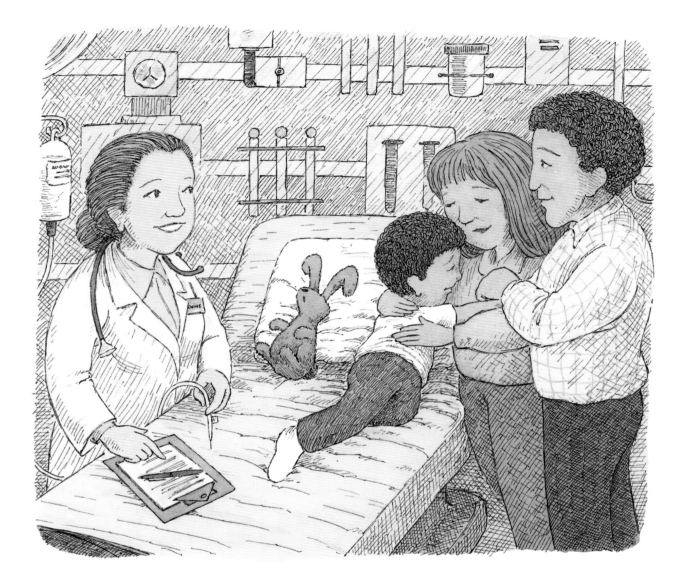

Harry's mom cuddled Harry for a little while and explained that Dr. Meadows wouldn't give him an IV if he didn't need it. Dr. Meadows told him the needle part would feel like a sharp pinch, but it would only be in his arm for a few seconds. The part that stayed in his arm would be a soft plastic tube that let the water go into his body, and it wouldn't hurt at all.

Dr. Meadows suggested that Harry's mom to tell him a story to help him think about something else when she put in the IV.

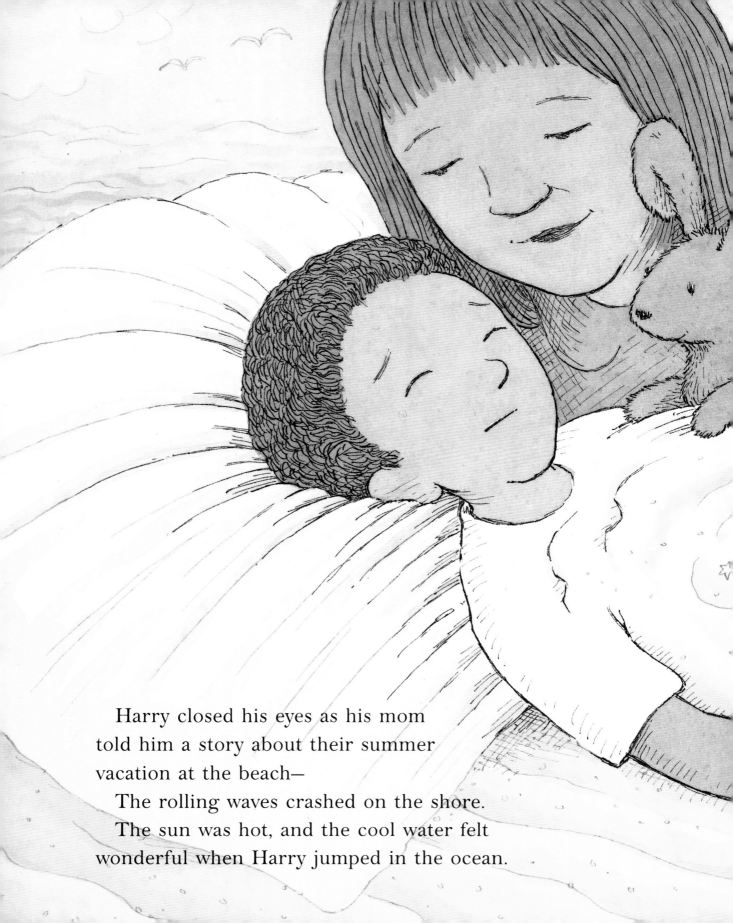

Harry closed his eyes as his mom
told him a story about their summer
vacation at the beach—
    The rolling waves crashed on the shore.
    The sun was hot, and the cool water felt
wonderful when Harry jumped in the ocean.

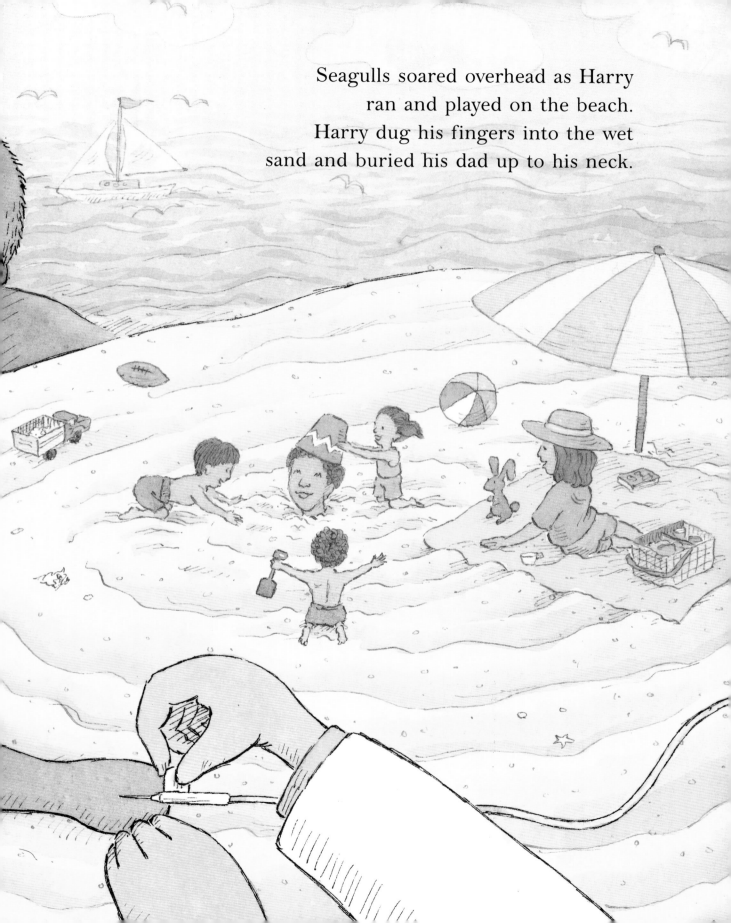

Seagulls soared overhead as Harry
ran and played on the beach.
Harry dug his fingers into the wet
sand and buried his dad up to his neck.

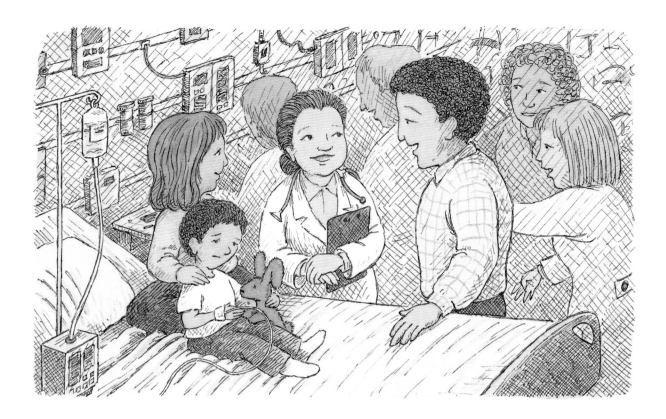

By the time Harry's mom was done with the story, Dr. Meadows had finished putting in the IV. The needle did hurt a little bit, just like she said it would, but it wasn't that bad. She taped his arm to a plastic board so the IV wouldn't fall out. It felt sort of stiff to Harry because he couldn't move his wrist, but it didn't hurt him at all.

Dr. Meadows talked to Harry and his parents. She said she wanted Harry to rest at the hospital for a day or two. That way they could be sure he was feeling better. Harry didn't like the idea of staying at the hospital, but he was glad that his mom said she'd stay with him the whole time. He closed his eyes and went to sleep.

When Harry woke up from his nap, his mom was sitting in a chair next to his bed, but his dad wasn't there.

"Where's Dad?" Harry cried.

"Oh honey, he had to go home to be with your brother and sister. Grandma came over to watch them when we brought you to the hospital, but she needed to leave. Dad will be back tomorrow, but remember, I'll be with you all night."

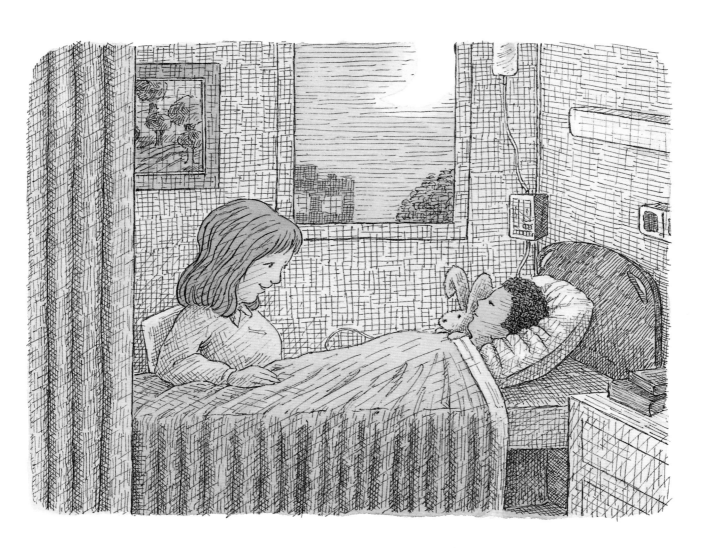

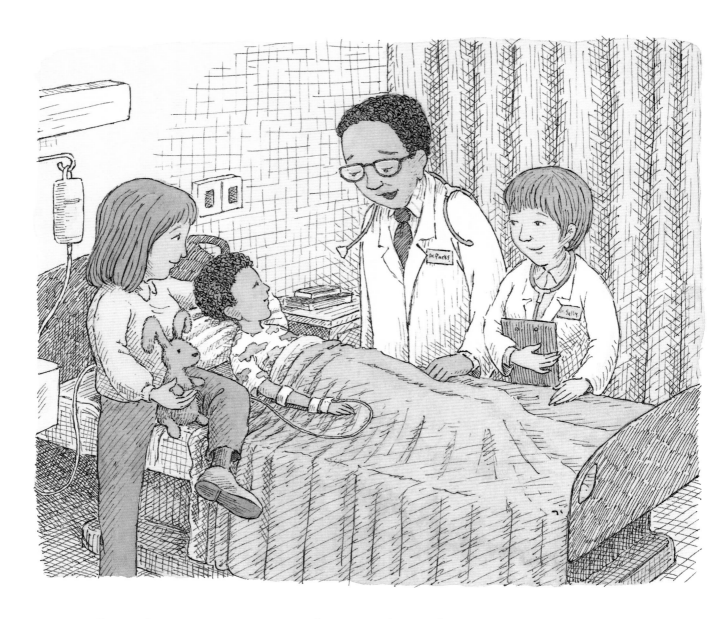

Just then, two new people came into the room.

"Hi, Harry. My name is Dr. Parks, and this is Sally Jenkins. Sally is a student doctor. She'll be working with me to make you better."

Harry didn't like having to meet so many people. Everything kept changing. He was glad that Mom was there. Especially when she stroked his hair and scratched Barney's ears.

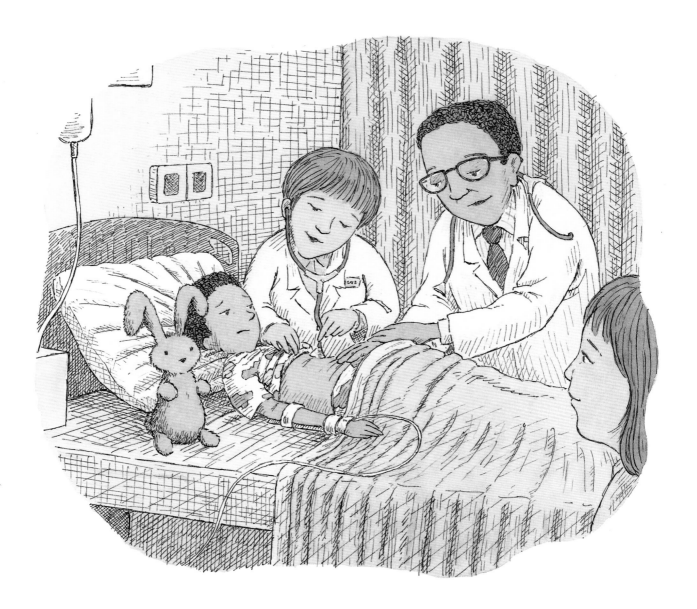

"They aren't going to give me another IV, are they?"
Harry asked his mom.

"No, sweetie, the one you have is working fine."

Harry tried to be brave and lay still while the new
doctors listened to his heart and pushed on his
tummy. Even though he did what the doctors asked,
Harry wasn't feeling very brave.

That night Harry had trouble falling asleep. His mom asked him what was wrong. Harry said he was worried that he got sick because he hit his brother when they were fighting the other day. Harry's mom kissed him on the forehead and said that no one gets sick because of something they did or didn't do. She said it was no one's fault if a person gets sick. Harry smiled and closed his eyes.

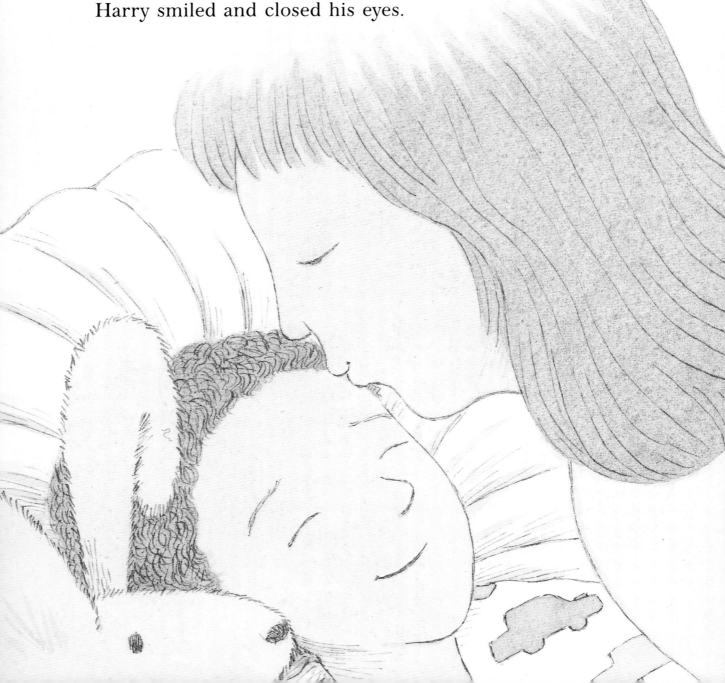

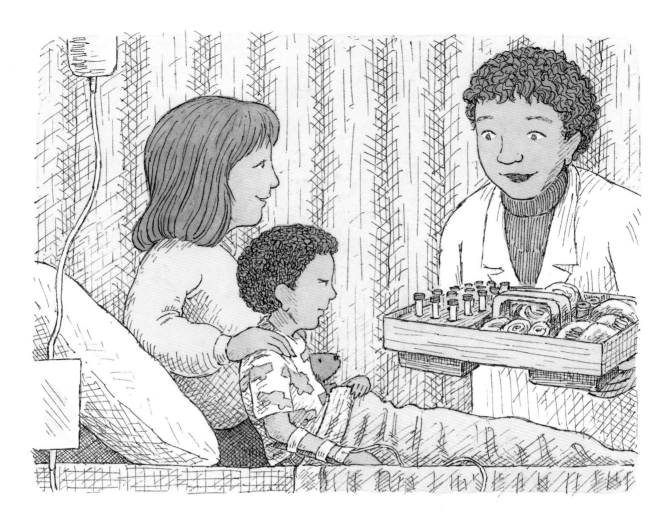

When Harry woke up the next morning, another new person was standing at the foot of his bed. He was carrying a tray filled with tubes. "Oh no," Harry thought.

"Hi, Harry. My name is DJ. I'm here to do a blood test."

Harry got nervous and hugged Barney tightly.

"This is just a finger poke, Harry, so it will only hurt for a second."

Harry believed DJ because Dr. Walker had given him finger pokes in his office and they didn't hurt that much. But Harry was tired and didn't want anyone else bothering him.

When DJ left, Harry felt thirsty and the nurse gave him a cup of juice.

He just took a few sips and then he threw up. His tummy began to hurt a lot, so the nurse called Dr. Parks. After he checked Harry, Dr. Parks said he wanted to get an X-ray of Harry's tummy to see what was making it hurt so much.

Harry had never heard of an X-ray. "Will it hurt?"

"No, Harry. An X-ray is a special picture that lets us see inside your body. The one we use for tummy aches is called a CAT scan. The machine that takes the picture looks a little funny, sort of like a great big donut, but it won't hurt you."

Harry wondered what cats were doing in the hospital, but Dr. Parks told him CAT scan was just a funny name that doctors used for the machine.

Harry's nurse took him to the X-ray room in a red wagon. They had to go slowly, but the nurse said Harry could pretend he was a racecar driver speeding around the track. He made engine sounds and waved to the other kids as he went by.

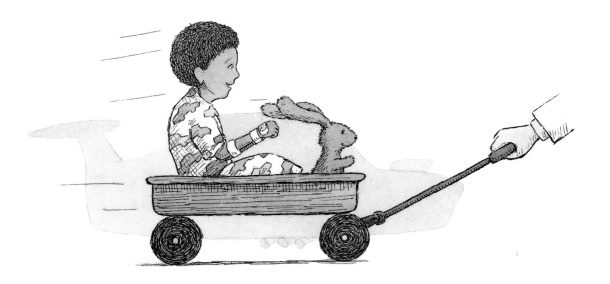

Harry thought it would be scary inside the CAT scan machine, but there was plenty of room and the nurse talked to him the entire time.

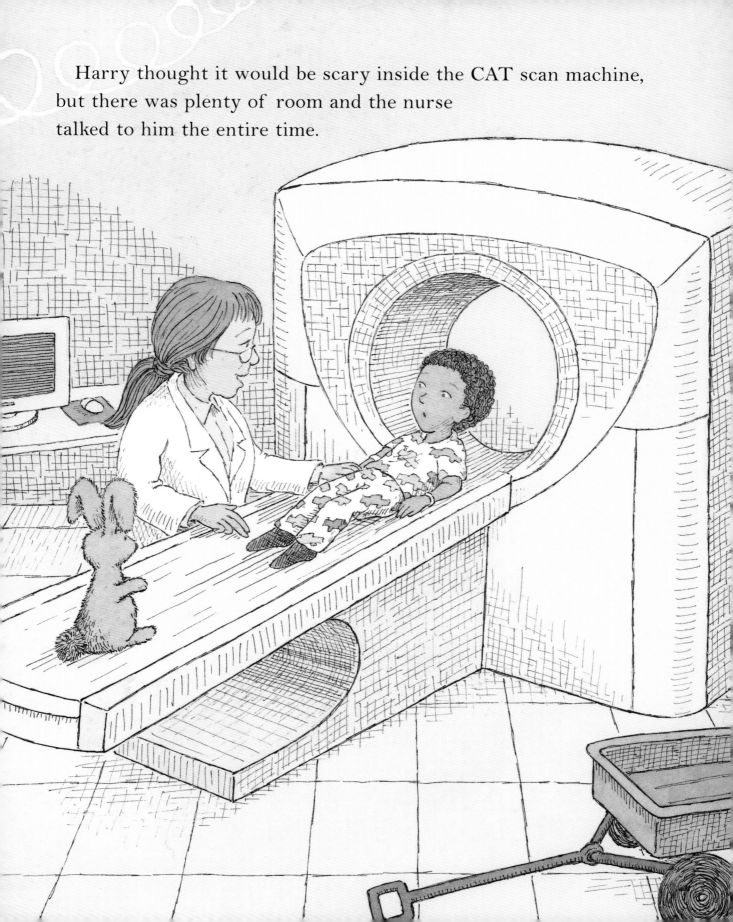

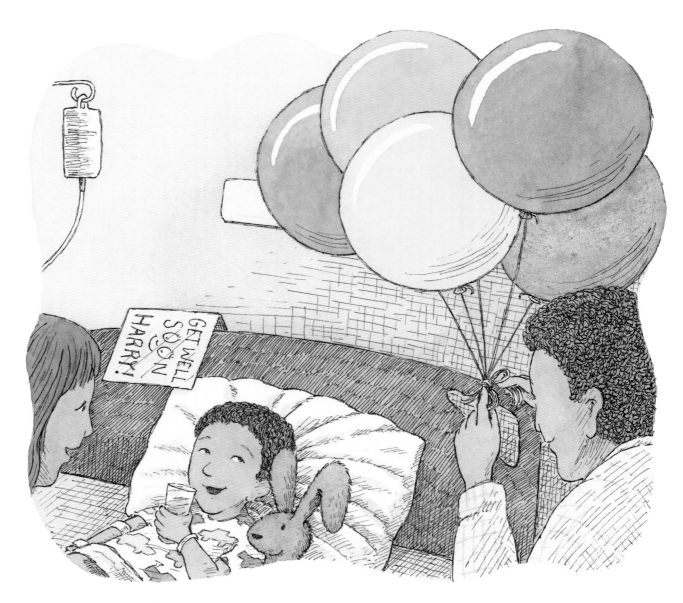

When Harry's CAT scan was done, Dr. Parks said his tummy was okay.

A few hours later, Harry's dad came back with balloons and a get-well card from his brother and sister. Harry liked that!

Harry was thirsty again. This time he drank some apple juice and didn't throw up. Harry liked that even more!

Harry slept for a little while and woke up when a nice woman named Ellie came to see him. Ellie told Harry that she was a child life specialist. Her job was to play with kids to help them with their feelings about being in the hospital.

"How are you today, Harry?"

"My tummy doesn't hurt anymore."

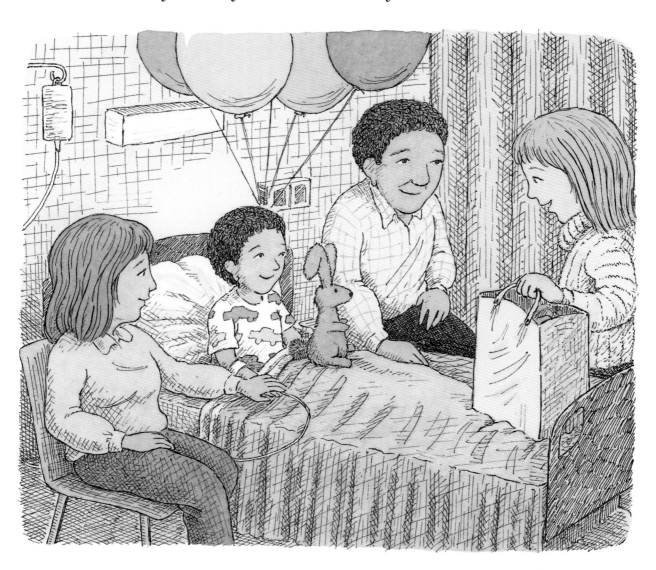

"That's great! I have some hospital toys that I wanted to show you. I've got a stethoscope, a thermometer, a light, and even an IV. Lots of kids like to use them on one of our dolls named Dr. Bob. Would you like to try them out?"

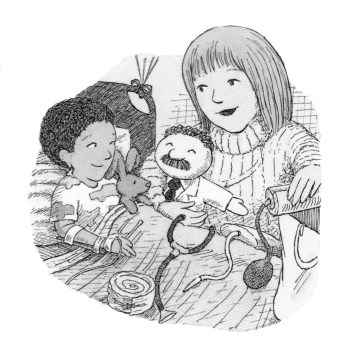

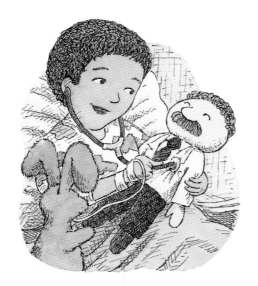

Harry smiled and began to give Dr. Bob a checkup. After he listened to his heart with the stethoscope and felt his tummy, Harry reached for the IV.

"Most kids don't like getting needles because they're afraid they might hurt," said Ellie.

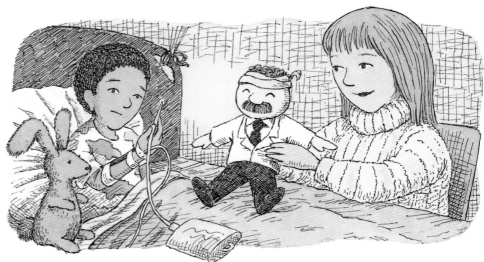

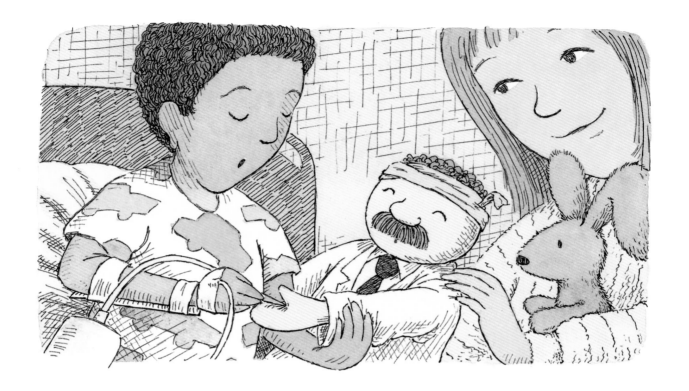

Harry stuck the needle in Dr. Bob's arm and said,
"I'm sorry, Dr. Bob, but you're very sick, and you need to
get an IV. It will make you feel better."

Ellie talked for Dr. Bob. "Then how come it hurts?"

Ellie could see that Harry liked playing with the hospital
instruments. She told him that Dr. Bob has gotten lots of
needles, since most kids like giving him an IV.

Harry played with his doctor tools for a long time.
Not only did Dr. Bob get an IV, but he also needed a blood
test, and he had to eat chicken soup when he really wanted
a slice of pepperoni pizza.

Dr. Parks stopped by when Ellie left. He said Harry could
go home in the morning if he didn't throw up anymore.

That brought a big smile to Harry's face.

Harry had a good night's sleep and woke up feeling much much better. He even got to eat pancakes! After breakfast, the nurse came in to see him.

"Harry, I have good news. Dr. Parks said you're ready to go home. I came in to take out your IV."

"Is it going to hurt when you take it out?"

"No, Harry. It comes out so fast that it will feel like a tiny pinch."

"Do I get a Band-Aid when you're done?"

"Absolutely!"

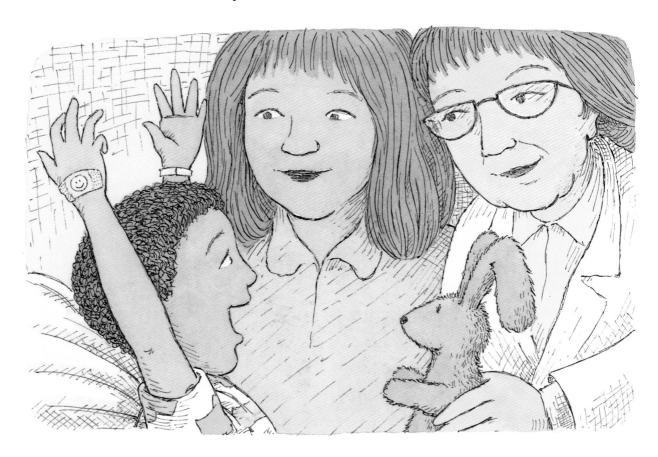

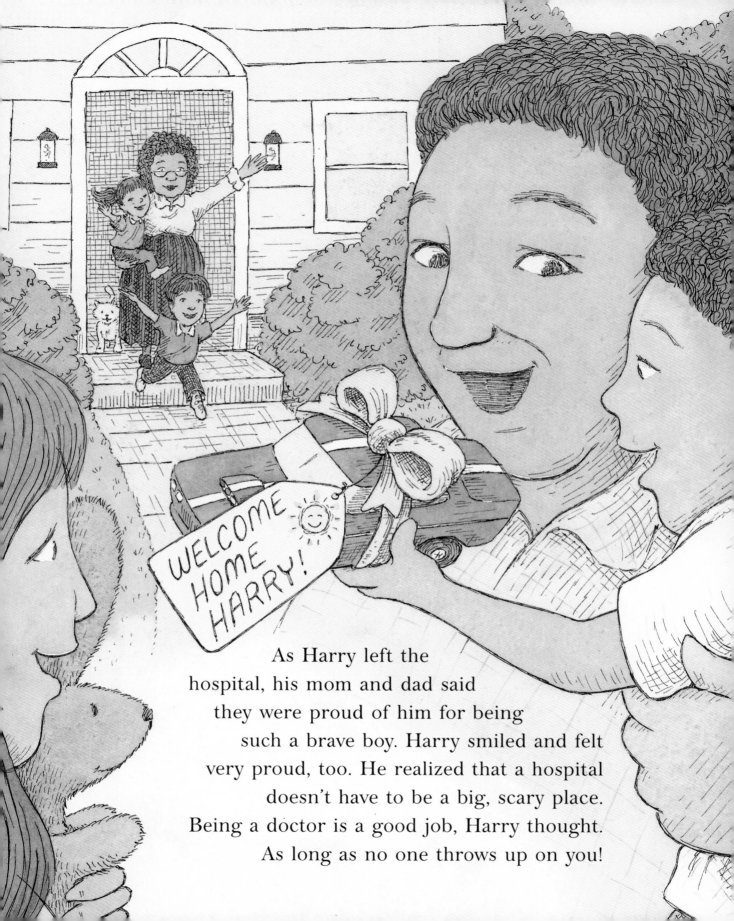

As Harry left the hospital, his mom and dad said they were proud of him for being such a brave boy. Harry smiled and felt very proud, too. He realized that a hospital doesn't have to be a big, scary place. Being a doctor is a good job, Harry thought. As long as no one throws up on you!

WELCOME HOME HARRY!

Note to Parents

by Virginia Shiller, Ph.D.

Hospitals can be scary places, even for grown-ups. The often overwhelming setting of the hospital can exacerbate a sick child's feelings of vulnerability and anxiety. Dealing with a steady stream of new faces—doctors, nurses, and other support staff—is itself unnerving. Add to that strange and unfamiliar noises coming from big machines; uncomfortable probing; and the sight of many patients with a variety of ailments makes for a scene that will frighten the hardiest of children!

You can provide a critical role in supporting your child as he navigates the many challenges of a hospital visit. If you have the opportunity to read this book before a trip to the emergency room or a hospital stay, you and your child will have the luxury of knowing about and discussing in advance many of the experiences that await you.

If, as often happens, you had to speed to the hospital with little warning, it's not too late to get help from this book! You can use it to help your child talk about the scary experiences—reviewing and retelling frightening experiences helps us all feel less vulnerable.

How You Can Help Your Child

The verbal and non-verbal signals you give to your child as she confronts frightening situations can either diminish or heighten her anxiety. Upon arriving at the hospital, your child will inevitably anxiously wonder: How dangerous is this place? Part of the answer to this question comes from how you, the parents, are reacting. If you do your best

to remain calm and reassuring, your child's anxiety can move down a notch.

But what about your own fears associated with hospitals and your child being sick? You shouldn't ignore your personal feelings. If possible, ask a friend or relative to join you for support. If that's not possible, simply step aside, call a friend and talk to her about what's going on. Sometimes, you need to take care of yourself to be able to care for your child. Keep in mind that while you need to listen to your feelings, it is best if you don't communicate your fears to your child who is (most likely) more frightened than you!

Other Practical Things You Can Do

- At the hospital, give your child information that will help him understand what is happening. Knowledge is power, and simply explaining the function of medical equipment can start to make a hospital feel somewhat less frightening. At home afterwards, encourage your child to talk about his hospital stay and use the illustrations in this book to evoke memories. Talking about things he remembers can help him develop a sense of mastery over the experience.
- Don't hesitate to speak up about what might help your child feel comfortable. Make suggestions to the medical staff that could add some comfort or familiarity. In the story, Harry's mother asks the doctor to first give a checkup to Harry's favorite stuffed animal, just as Harry's pediatrician typically would

do during office visits. It makes Harry feel more "at home." Most doctors will welcome such suggestions. (If you missed this step, a simple "Gee, I wish we had asked the doctor to give Barney a check-up, too" will communicate empathy and caring to your child.)

- Don't overdo efforts to encourage your child to face challenges bravely. It's best to strive for a balance of validating your child's scary feelings and commending him for courageously coping. Certainly, congratulate her when she rises to challenges. Show your pride through praise or a pat on the back. But, if your child is looking very frightened, let her know that you understand that what's going on is scary. Then, tell her you're going to do your best to make things as comfortable as possible.

Relaxation and Visualization Techniques

Harry Goes to the Hospital illustrates how you can help your child relax while undergoing stressful procedures. While an IV is being inserted, the doctor encourages Harry's mother to tell him a story. Harry closes his eyes, and his mother describes in detail experiences they shared during their summer beach vacation. As she tells the story, Harry visualizes rolling waves, hot sun, soaring seagulls, and wet sand.

Stories encouraging your child to relax can be especially helpful if they involve vivid and pleasurable scenes. If you use a slow, soft, soothing voice to describe the scenes, this technique can be especially powerful. (And in the process of gently describing scenes, you may find yourself relaxing, too!)

Tailoring the story to your child's unique interests may also maximize the story's distractive value. If your child loves Star Wars adventures, you might take one of her favorite characters on a space flight. A dinosaur fan may be captivated by a story of a time capsule trip back to the age of dinosaurs.

Play as Therapy

The story also introduces the idea that simple play activities can diminish fears and increase a child's sense of mastery. Ellie, a hospital child life specialist, visits Harry and invites him to play with toy medical instruments. How exciting to become the one using the stethoscope or inserting needles!

By allowing children to actively be in charge rather than being the passive recipient of painful procedures, play can help children put scary experiences behind them.

Your child may want to play out the hospital experiences after you return home. Providing him with props such as a toy medical kit is helpful. Don't try to direct this play; the goal is for him to feel in charge.

Also, don't be surprised if he begins experimenting using medical instruments in different ways: An IV could be inserted in the arm, the leg, and maybe even a doll's ear. If you're game, volunteer to be the patient, and wince and whimper as he gleefully pricks you with play needles! We all feel better when we can find a humorous side to a scary and sometimes painful experience.

When to Do More

In most cases, a trip to the hospital is a stressful experience you can help your child put in perspective. However, if your child's experiences were particularly painful or frightening, or if she has a medical problem that will require further hospitalizations, keep an eye on her behavior. If there are signs of anxiety, such as sleep problems, tummy aches, or clinginess, or if she either becomes obsessed with hospital play or avoids any reminders of the hospital, it may be wise to consult a professional.

— *VIRGINIA SHILLER, PH.D., is a clinical psychologist in private practice in New Haven, Connecticut, and a Lecturer at the Yale Child Study Center. She is the author, with MEG SCHNEIDER, of* Rewards for Kids! Ready-to-Use Charts and Reward Activities for Positive Parenting.

About the Author

HOWARD J. BENNETT, M.D., practices pediatrics in Washington, D.C., and lives in Maryland with his wife and two children. He is the author of *Lions Aren't Scared of Shots, It Hurts When I Poop!* and *Waking Up Dry: A Guide to Help Children Overcome Bedwetting.* Dr. Bennett is also a clinical professor of pediatrics at the George Washington University School of Medicine and a member of the Community Advisory Staff at the Children's National Medical Center. He maintains a website (www.wakingupdry.com) where he posts information related to bedwetting.

About the Illustrator

M.S. (MICHAEL) WEBER is a graduate of the Art Institute of Chicago. His illustrations appear in children's books and magazines, and online at Magickeys.com. "I look upon children as a new frontier," he says, "because if children are well influenced through their parents, education, and literature, the chances of our world becoming a better place will improve. This is why I illustrate children's stories." He lives in Chicago with his family.